SAMANTHA PETEREIN

The Modern Herbalist's Guide

30 Days to Healing and Harmony

To my family–
For your endless love, patience, and unwavering support. You are
my foundation, my inspiration, and the heart of everything I do.

Contents

Introduction

Welcome to The Modern Herbalist's Guide: 30 Days to Healing and Harmony.

In today's fast-paced world, finding balance and connection to ourselves and nature has become increasingly difficult. The Modern Herbalist's Guide is designed to help you slow down, reconnect with the healing power of herbs, and establish a meaningful daily self-care practice. Over the next 30 days, you'll explore herbs that nurture your body, mind, and spirit, while cultivating mindful rituals that bring balance and peace into your life.

Each day in this journey, you will:

- Meet an Herb: Learn about an herb's healing properties and how to incorporate it into your daily routine.
- Practice a Ritual: Engage in a self-care ritual that allows you to work with the herb in a tangible way.
- Meditate Mindfully: Follow a short, guided meditation designed to help you reflect on the energy of the herb and its healing properties.
- Journal for Reflection: Use the journaling prompt to deepen your self-awareness and understanding of the healing

journey.

This is not just a guide—it's a commitment to yourself. Over the next 30 days, you'll create space for healing, reflection, and mindful self-care. Take it one day at a time, and allow yourself the grace to grow.

I

Medical Disclaimer

A Journey Through Herbal History and Healing

Herbs have been a part of human healing traditions for thousands of years, spanning cultures and continents. From the ancient Egyptians to traditional Chinese medicine practitioners, herbs have played a vital role in treating ailments, restoring balance, and promoting well-being. Today, herbs continue to be a source of healing and nourishment, offering a gentle yet powerful way to care for the body, mind, and spirit.

Herbalism, the practice of using plants for their medicinal properties, is rooted in our connection to the earth. Every culture around the world has developed its own unique approach to herbal healing. Some of the earliest records date back to 3000 BCE in Egypt, where herbs were used in medicine and even embalming practices. In Ayurvedic medicine, herbs like turmeric and ashwagandha have been used for thousands of years to promote health and longevity. In traditional Chinese medicine, herbs are often paired with acupuncture and other holistic therapies to bring balance to the body's energy (qi).

While the ways in which we use herbs have evolved, the essence remains the same—plants have the ability to heal, restore, and bring balance. Today, herbs are used in many forms, including:

- Teas: Infusing herbs in hot water to extract their healing properties.
- Tinctures: Concentrated herbal extracts made by steeping herbs in alcohol or glycerin.
- Essential Oils: Highly concentrated oils extracted from plants, often used in aromatherapy.
- Salves and Balms: Topical herbal preparations used to soothe and heal the skin.
- Aromatherapy: The use of essential oils for their emotional, physical, and spiritual benefits through scent.

Herbs and Essential Oils: Beyond the Cup of Tea

In addition to consuming herbs in teas or tinctures, essential oils are an effective and accessible way to benefit from the healing properties of plants. Aromatherapy, the practice of using plant oils for emotional and physical well-being, has roots in ancient Greece and Rome, where oils were used for healing, religious ceremonies, and even in everyday hygiene.

Essential oils, like lavender for relaxation, peppermint for energy, and eucalyptus for respiratory support, work by interacting with the limbic system in the brain, which regulates emotions and memory. By diffusing these oils or applying them topically (diluted), you can enhance your emotional and physical well-being.

As we journey through the next 30 days, you'll explore herbs in various forms—teas, essential oils, baths, and more—incorporating them into your daily rituals. Whether you're seeking to relieve stress, improve sleep, or find more energy, you'll learn how to harness the power of herbs in a way that feels natural and accessible.

Day 1: Chamomile (Matricaria chamomilla)

Herb of the Day: Chamomile

Chamomile is a gentle yet powerful herb known for its calming and anti-inflammatory properties. It soothes the nervous system, reduces anxiety, and promotes restful sleep. Chamomile is ideal for those seeking peace and relaxation in moments of stress or restlessness.

- Healing Properties: Calms anxiety, aids sleep, soothes digestive discomfort, reduces inflammation.
- How to Use: Brew a cup of chamomile tea in the evening, use chamomile essential oil in a diffuser, or add dried chamomile to a warm bath.

Guided Meditation:

- Close your eyes and take a deep breath in, feeling the air fill your lungs, and exhale slowly. Picture yourself surrounded by a field of chamomile flowers. With each inhale, imagine the calming energy of the flowers filling your body, easing tension, and bringing peace. As you exhale, release any worries or stress. Focus on the idea of rest and restoration, allowing the herb's energy to soothe your mind and body. Sit with this peaceful imagery for a few minutes, breathing deeply.

Daily Ritual:

- Chamomile Tea Ritual: Brew a cup of chamomile tea in the evening before bed. As you sip, focus on the warmth of the tea, the scent of the chamomile, and how your body relaxes with each sip. This is your time to unwind and let go of the day.

Alternative Uses:

- Chamomile Essential Oil: Diffuse chamomile essential oil in your bedroom or living space for a calming atmosphere. You can also add a few drops of the essential oil to a carrier oil and apply it to your temples or wrists for relaxation during stressful moments.
- Herbal Bath: Add dried chamomile flowers to a warm bath for a soothing, full-body relaxation experience. Chamomile's anti-inflammatory properties can also help soothe irritated skin.

- Chamomile Compress: Brew a strong chamomile tea, let it cool, then soak a cloth in the tea and apply it as a compress to tired eyes or irritated skin for a calming effect.

II

Journaling Prompt:

What areas of your life feel most stressful right now, and how can you introduce more calm into those moments? Reflect on how chamomile's energy might help you find balance.

Day 2: Lavender (Lavandula angustifolia)

H erb of the Day: Lavender

Lavender is a well-known herb celebrated for its calming and soothing properties. It helps ease anxiety, promote restful sleep, and can be used to treat minor skin irritations. Lavender is widely available and versatile, making it an excellent choice for beginners.

- Healing Properties: Calms the nervous system, supports restful sleep, reduces stress, and soothes irritated skin.
- How to Use: Lavender can be used in teas, tinctures, essential oils, or added to baths. You can also use dried lavender to make herbal sachets to place under your pillow.

Guided Meditation:

- Sit comfortably and close your eyes. Imagine yourself walking through a field of lavender, the scent of the flowers surrounding you, bringing peace with every breath. Inhale deeply and feel the calming energy of lavender wash over you. As you exhale, release any tension from your body. Repeat this visualization for several minutes, allowing lavender's essence to calm your mind and spirit.

Daily Ritual:

- Lavender Essential Oil Diffusion: Add a few drops of lavender essential oil to a diffuser in your bedroom in the evening. As the scent fills the air, focus on your breathing, inhaling the calming aroma and allowing it to relax your body and mind before sleep.

Alternative Uses:

- Topical Use: Add a few drops of lavender essential oil to a carrier oil (like coconut oil) and apply to your temples or wrists when you're feeling stressed or anxious.
- Herbal Bath: Add dried lavender to a warm bath for a soothing, skin-nourishing soak.

III

Journaling Prompt:

What areas of your life feel out of balance? How can you bring more peace and relaxation into those moments? Reflect on how lavender's calming properties can help you create more space for rest.

Day 3: Peppermint (Mentha piperita)

Herb of the Day: Peppermint

Peppermint is an invigorating and refreshing herb, known for its ability to support digestion, increase focus, and relieve headaches. Its cooling properties make it an excellent herb for both physical and mental clarity.

- Healing Properties: Supports digestion, reduces headaches, increases energy, and clears mental fog.
- How to Use: Peppermint can be enjoyed as a tea, used in tinctures, or inhaled as an essential oil for an instant boost of energy and focus.

Guided Meditation:

- Close your eyes and take a deep breath in, imagining the crisp, cool scent of peppermint filling your lungs. As you inhale, feel your mind becoming sharper and clearer. With each exhale, release any mental fog or sluggishness. Focus on the idea of clarity and energy, using peppermint's fresh energy to renew your focus.

Daily Ritual:

- Peppermint Tea for Clarity: Brew a cup of peppermint tea in the morning or midday. As you sip, focus on the refreshing taste and how it energizes your body and mind. Use this time to set your intentions for the day or reset your energy during a midday break.

Alternative Uses:

- Aromatherapy: Inhale peppermint essential oil directly from the bottle or apply a few drops to a diffuser for a quick burst of energy and mental clarity.
- Topical Use: Dilute peppermint essential oil in a carrier oil and apply it to your temples to relieve tension headaches.

IV

Journaling Prompt:

How can you create more clarity in your life? What is clouding your mind, and how can you clear away distractions? Reflect on peppermint's energizing properties and how they might help you regain focus.

Day 4: Calendula (Calendula officinalis)

H erb of the Day: Calendula

Calendula is known for its skin-healing properties. It helps soothe irritated skin, reduce inflammation, and can be used to promote wound healing. This gentle herb is great for topical use, making it perfect for beginners looking to incorporate natural skin care into their routine.

- Healing Properties: Soothes irritated skin, promotes healing of cuts and scrapes, reduces inflammation.
- How to Use: Calendula can be used in oils, salves, or teas. Apply calendula-infused oil to the skin or use it in a salve for cuts and scrapes.

Guided Meditation:

- Sit in a quiet space and close your eyes. Picture a bright orange calendula flower blooming in the sun. Imagine the flower's vibrant energy spreading through your body, bringing healing warmth and light to any areas that feel tense or sore. Inhale deeply, visualizing this healing energy, and exhale, letting go of any physical or emotional discomfort.

Daily Ritual:

- Calendula Skin Salve: If you have a calendula salve or oil, apply it to any areas of dry or irritated skin today. As you massage it in, focus on the healing energy of the plant, thanking your body for its ability to heal.

Alternative Uses:

- Herbal Bath: Add calendula flowers to a warm bath for a soothing, skin-healing soak.
- Calendula Tea: Drink calendula tea to promote internal healing and reduce inflammation.

V

Journaling Prompt:

What areas of your life feel like they need healing?
How can you nourish yourself more
deeply—physically, emotionally, or spiritually?
Reflect on calendula's healing energy and how you
can apply it to your own journey.

Day 5: Lemon Balm (Melissa officinalis)

Herb of the Day: Lemon Balm

Lemon balm is a calming herb that supports emotional balance, reduces anxiety, and can help lift your mood. Its bright, lemony scent is uplifting and refreshing, making it a favorite for those seeking emotional support.

- Healing Properties: Reduces anxiety, lifts mood, calms the nervous system.
- How to Use: Lemon balm can be used in teas, tinctures, or as an essential oil for its calming effects.

Guided Meditation:

- Take a deep breath in and imagine the fresh, citrus scent of lemon balm filling your senses. As you breathe in, feel a sense of calm and happiness wash over you. Picture a bright, sunny day, with a gentle breeze and warmth surrounding you. Let this visualization lift your mood and calm your mind.

Daily Ritual:

- Lemon Balm Tea for Emotional Balance: Brew a cup of lemon balm tea in the afternoon. As you sip, focus on the soothing, uplifting qualities of the herb. Reflect on how it calms your emotions and helps you find a sense of peace.

Alternative Uses:

- Aromatherapy: Use lemon balm essential oil in a diffuser to create a calming atmosphere in your home.
- Topical Use: Make a lemon balm-infused oil and apply it to your skin for its soothing effects.

VI

Journaling Prompt:

How can you bring more emotional balance into your life? What is currently causing you stress or anxiety, and how can you gently ease those feelings? Reflect on how lemon balm can support your emotional well-being.

Day 6: Eucalyptus (Eucalyptus globulus)

Herb of the Day: Eucalyptus

Eucalyptus is a powerful herb known for its ability to clear the respiratory system and provide mental clarity. It is commonly used in essential oils and salves to soothe colds and congestion, making it a go-to herb for respiratory support and fresh energy.

- Healing Properties: Clears the respiratory system, boosts mental clarity, reduces inflammation.
- How to Use: Eucalyptus can be used in essential oil form for aromatherapy, added to baths for respiratory relief, or applied topically in salves.

Guided Meditation:

- Close your eyes and take a deep breath, imagining the fresh, crisp scent of eucalyptus clearing your lungs and mind. As you inhale, feel the cool air move through your body, bringing clarity and energy. With each exhale, release any mental fog or congestion. Allow yourself to sit with this feeling of openness and freshness, using the energy of eucalyptus to cleanse and clear your mind and body.

Daily Ritual:

- Eucalyptus Steam Inhalation: Boil water and pour it into a large bowl. Add a few drops of eucalyptus essential oil or dried eucalyptus leaves. Cover your head with a towel and lean over the bowl, inhaling the steam deeply. This practice can clear the respiratory system and open your airways, especially if you're feeling congested.

Alternative Uses:

- Aromatherapy: Diffuse eucalyptus essential oil in your home or workspace for mental clarity and to clear the airways.
- Topical Application: Dilute eucalyptus essential oil in a carrier oil and massage into the chest or temples to soothe congestion or relieve muscle tension.
- Bath Soak: Add eucalyptus oil or leaves to a warm bath for a refreshing, invigorating experience that clears the sinuses.

VII

Journaling Prompt:

*How can you bring more clarity into your life, both
mentally and physically?
Reflect on any areas where you feel "stuck" or
congested, and how eucalyptus can help you clear
space for new energy.*

Day 7: Rosemary (Rosmarinus officinalis)

H erb of the Day: Rosemary

Rosemary is a stimulating herb that sharpens memory, increases focus, and supports circulation. It has been used for centuries to enhance mental clarity and is often associated with remembrance and protection.

- Healing Properties: Sharpens memory, improves focus, supports circulation, relieves headaches.
- How to Use: Rosemary can be used in teas, as an essential oil, or in culinary dishes to enhance both flavor and mental clarity.

Guided Meditation:

- Sit comfortably and close your eyes. Visualize a bright, aromatic rosemary bush growing in the sunlight. With each inhale, feel the energy of rosemary sharpening your mind and bringing clarity. As you exhale, let go of distractions or mental clutter. Use rosemary's stimulating energy to focus on your goals and intentions for the day.

Daily Ritual:

- Rosemary Infusion for Focus: Brew a cup of rosemary tea in the morning or afternoon when you need mental clarity. As you drink, focus on how the herb sharpens your senses and brings energy to your body. Use this time to center yourself before starting a task that requires focus.

Alternative Uses:

- Aromatherapy: Inhale rosemary essential oil directly or diffuse it in your workspace to improve focus and mental clarity.
- Hair Rinse: Create a rosemary infusion by steeping fresh or dried rosemary in hot water. Let it cool, then rinse your hair with it to stimulate scalp circulation and support hair growth.
- Culinary Use: Add rosemary to your meals—whether in soups, roasted vegetables, or bread—for both flavor and cognitive benefits.

VIII

Journaling Prompt:

What are your current goals, and how can you sharpen your focus to achieve them? Reflect on how rosemary's energy of clarity and remembrance can help you stay focused and on track.

Day 8: Ginger (Zingiber officinale)

Herb of the Day: Ginger

Ginger is a warming and invigorating herb that stimulates circulation, aids digestion, and relieves nausea. Known for its spicy and comforting flavor, ginger is often used in teas and culinary dishes to bring warmth and energy to the body.

- Healing Properties: Stimulates circulation, aids digestion, relieves nausea, reduces inflammation.
- How to Use: Ginger can be used in teas, tinctures, or added to food for its warming properties and health benefits.

Guided Meditation:

- Sit quietly and close your eyes. Picture a warming fire in your belly, gently radiating warmth throughout your body. With each breath, feel the energy of ginger warming you from the inside out, bringing vitality and comfort. As you exhale, release any coldness or stagnation. Allow the warmth of ginger to fill you with energy and motivation.

Daily Ritual:

• Ginger Tea for Warming Energy: Brew a cup of fresh ginger tea by slicing a few pieces of ginger root and steeping them in hot water. As you drink, feel the warmth spreading through your body. Use this tea to wake up your senses in the morning or to soothe digestion after a meal.

Alternative Uses:

• Culinary Use: Add fresh or powdered ginger to your meals to stimulate digestion and circulation. Ginger is especially delicious in soups, stir-fries, or baked goods.
• Topical Use: Make a ginger compress by steeping fresh ginger in hot water, soaking a cloth in the infusion, and applying it to areas of the body that need warmth and circulation (like stiff muscles or cold hands).
• Essential Oil: Add a few drops of ginger essential oil to a carrier oil and massage into areas of tension for warmth and relief.

IX

Journaling Prompt:

Where in your life do you need more warmth or motivation? Reflect on how ginger's energy of warmth and movement can help you move through areas of stagnation and bring vitality.

Day 9: Sage (Salvia officinalis)

erb of the Day: Sage

Sage is a cleansing and protective herb, often used to clear negative energy and support respiratory health. It has been used in spiritual practices for centuries to purify spaces and the body, making it a powerful herb for both physical and energetic cleansing.

- Healing Properties: Clears negative energy, supports respiratory health, reduces inflammation.
- How to Use: Sage can be used in smudging rituals to purify spaces, brewed into a tea for its respiratory benefits, or burned as incense.

Guided Meditation:

- Close your eyes and take a deep breath, imagining the cleansing scent of sage filling the air around you. As you inhale, feel the purifying energy of the herb clearing away any negative thoughts or stagnant energy. Exhale, letting go of anything that no longer serves you. Visualize yourself surrounded by a protective light, created by the energy of sage.

Daily Ritual:

• Sage Smudging Ritual: Light a sage bundle or a stick of dried sage, allowing the smoke to rise. Move the smoke around your body or your space, focusing on areas that feel energetically heavy or stagnant. As you do this, repeat an affirmation of cleansing and protection.

Alternative Uses:

• Sage Tea: Brew a cup of sage tea to support respiratory health and reduce inflammation, especially during cold or flu season.
• Aromatherapy: Use sage essential oil in a diffuser to purify the air and create a calming, protective atmosphere in your home.
• Topical Use: Make a sage-infused oil to massage into the skin for its anti-inflammatory and antimicrobial properties.

X

Journaling Prompt:

What negative energy or habits do you need to release? Reflect on how you can create more protection and clarity in your life, using sage as a tool for cleansing both physically and energetically.

Day 10: Holy Basil (Tulsi) (Ocimum tenuiflorum)

Herb of the Day: Holy Basil

Holy Basil, also known as Tulsi, is revered in Ayurvedic medicine for its ability to reduce stress, support the immune system, and promote mental clarity. It's often called the "elixir of life" for its wide range of healing properties, including emotional and physical balance.

- Healing Properties: Reduces stress, boosts the immune system, supports mental clarity and emotional balance.
- How to Use: Holy Basil is most commonly consumed as tea, tincture, or in capsule form. It can also be used as an essential oil to reduce stress and promote clarity.

Guided Meditation:

- Sit quietly, close your eyes, and take a deep breath in. Imagine yourself surrounded by the calming energy of a

Holy Basil plant. With each inhale, feel the stress in your body slowly dissolve. As you exhale, let go of any emotional tension, allowing yourself to feel at peace. Focus on the theme of balance and clarity as Holy Basil brings harmony to your body and mind.

Daily Ritual:

- Holy Basil Tea for Emotional Balance: Brew a cup of Holy Basil tea and sip slowly, focusing on how it calms your body and reduces any lingering stress or anxiety. Let this ritual be a moment of peace in your day, bringing emotional balance and grounding.

Alternative Uses:

- Tincture: Add a dropper of Holy Basil tincture to your water or tea to promote emotional balance and stress reduction throughout the day.
- Aromatherapy: Use Holy Basil essential oil in a diffuser to create a calming atmosphere, especially when feeling overwhelmed.
- Topical Use: Dilute Holy Basil essential oil in a carrier oil and apply to your temples or wrists to promote relaxation.

XI

Journaling Prompt:

In what areas of your life do you feel out of balance?
How can you create more emotional harmony?
Reflect on how Holy Basil's balancing properties
might help you cultivate a sense of peace.

Day 11: Lemon (Citrus limon)

Herb of the Day: Lemon

Lemon is a bright, invigorating herb known for its detoxifying properties and ability to uplift the mood. Whether used in teas, essential oils, or culinary dishes, lemon brings a fresh energy to the body and mind, helping to cleanse and rejuvenate.

- Healing Properties: Uplifts mood, detoxifies the body, supports digestion, boosts immunity.
- How to Use: Lemon can be used in water or tea, as a culinary addition, or as an essential oil to uplift the spirit and cleanse the body.

Guided Meditation:

- Close your eyes and take a deep breath in, imagining the bright, citrusy scent of lemon filling your lungs. As you inhale, feel a sense of clarity and rejuvenation spread throughout your body. As you exhale, let go of any stagnant energy or tension. Focus on the theme of cleansing and renewal as you allow lemon's refreshing energy to wash over you.

Daily Ritual:

- Lemon Water for Detoxification: Start your morning with a glass of warm water with fresh lemon juice. As you drink, focus on the cleansing and detoxifying properties of the lemon, envisioning it clearing out any toxins from your body and bringing fresh energy to your day.

Alternative Uses:

- Aromatherapy: Diffuse lemon essential oil to uplift the spirit and create a fresh, clean atmosphere in your home.
- Topical Use: Add a few drops of lemon essential oil to a carrier oil and use it in a detoxifying massage, focusing on areas that feel heavy or congested.
- Culinary Use: Add fresh lemon to your meals or beverages to enhance flavor and promote digestive health.

XII

Journaling Prompt:

What areas of your life feel heavy or stagnant? How can you bring more clarity and lightness into those spaces? Reflect on how lemon's energy of renewal and detoxification can help you create fresh energy in your daily life.

Day 12: Dandelion (Taraxacum officinale)

Herb of the Day: Dandelion

Dandelion, often seen as a common weed, is a powerhouse of healing properties. It supports liver health, acts as a natural diuretic, and promotes detoxification. This humble plant is an excellent ally for anyone looking to cleanse and revitalize the body.

- Healing Properties: Supports liver health, promotes detoxification, acts as a natural diuretic.
- How to Use: Dandelion can be used in teas, tinctures, or added to salads. The leaves, roots, and flowers are all edible and medicinal.

Guided Meditation:

- Close your eyes and take a deep breath. Imagine a field of dandelions in the sunlight, their bright yellow flowers reflecting the energy of the sun. With each inhale, feel the detoxifying energy of the dandelion moving through your body, clearing out toxins and bringing vitality. As you exhale, let go of anything weighing you down, allowing the dandelion to renew your body and spirit.

Daily Ritual:

- Dandelion Root Tea for Liver Health: Brew a cup of dandelion root tea to support liver function and detoxification. As you sip, focus on the gentle, cleansing properties of the herb, allowing it to clear any physical or emotional stagnation from your system.

Alternative Uses:

- Culinary Use: Add fresh dandelion leaves to your salads for a bitter but nourishing detoxifying effect. Dandelion greens support digestion and liver health.
- Tincture: Take dandelion root tincture daily to gently cleanse the liver and support detoxification.
- Topical Use: Make a dandelion-infused oil to massage into areas of your body that feel stagnant or need support, such as your abdomen or feet.

XIII

Journaling Prompt:

What are you holding onto that no longer serves you? How can you release these toxins from your life—both physically and emotionally? Reflect on how dandelion's cleansing energy can support you in letting go and renewing your vitality.

Day 13: Marshmallow Root (Althaea officinalis)

Herb of the Day: Marshmallow Root

Marshmallow root is a soothing, mucilaginous herb that supports digestive health, soothes inflammation, and hydrates the body. Known for its ability to coat and protect mucous membranes, marshmallow is an excellent herb for anyone dealing with dryness, irritation, or inflammation.

- Healing Properties: Soothes inflammation, supports digestive health, hydrates the body.
- How to Use: Marshmallow root can be made into a cold infusion, used in teas, or taken as a tincture to soothe internal irritation and promote hydration.

Guided Meditation:

- Close your eyes and take a deep breath in, imagining a wave of soothing energy washing over you. With each inhale, feel the cooling, calming energy of marshmallow root filling your body. As you exhale, release any inflammation, irritation, or discomfort. Focus on the theme of healing and hydration as marshmallow root restores balance and peace to your body.

Daily Ritual:

· Marshmallow Root Cold Infusion: Make a cold infusion by soaking marshmallow root in cold water for several hours. As you drink the infusion, focus on how it soothes and hydrates your body, bringing relief to any areas of irritation or inflammation.

Alternative Uses:

· Topical Use: Use marshmallow-infused oil on irritated or dry skin for its soothing, hydrating properties.
· Digestive Support: Drink marshmallow tea regularly to soothe digestive discomfort or inflammation in the gut.
· Tincture: Take marshmallow root tincture to calm inflammation and promote internal healing.

XIV

Journaling Prompt:

What areas of your life feel inflamed or irritated? How can you bring more calm and soothing energy to these spaces? Reflect on how marshmallow root's soothing properties can help you restore peace and balance.

Day 14: Oatstraw (Avena sativa)

erb of the Day: Oatstraw

Oatstraw is a nourishing, calming herb that supports the nervous system, reduces stress, and promotes restful sleep. It's rich in vitamins and minerals, making it an excellent herb for overall wellness and long-term health support.

- Healing Properties: Nourishes the nervous system, reduces stress, supports restful sleep, and promotes overall wellness.
- How to Use: Oatstraw is best consumed as a tea or infusion, allowing the body to absorb its rich nutrients over time.

Guided Meditation:

- Close your eyes and take a deep breath in, imagining the soft, soothing energy of oatstraw wrapping around you like a blanket. With each inhale, feel the gentle nourishment of the herb filling your body, calming your mind and relaxing your muscles. As you exhale, release any stress or tension. Focus on the theme of nourishment as oatstraw supports your overall well-being.

Daily Ritual:

- Oatstraw Infusion for Nervous System Support: Make a nourishing infusion by steeping oatstraw in hot water for several hours. As you drink, focus on how the herb replenishes your nervous system, calming your mind and body.

Alternative Uses:

- Bath Soak: Add oatstraw to a warm bath for a soothing soak that calms the nervous system and hydrates the skin.
- Topical Use: Use oatstraw-infused oil on dry or irritated skin to provide deep nourishment and hydration.
- Herbal Hair Rinse: Rinse your hair with oatstraw tea to strengthen and nourish the hair and scalp.

XV

Journaling Prompt:

Where in your life do you need more nourishment, both physically and emotionally? How can you take better care of your body and mind? Reflect on how oatstraw's calming and nourishing properties can help you create more balance and well-being in your life.

Day 15: Red Clover (Trifolium pratense)

erb of the Day: Red Clover

Red clover is a gentle and nourishing herb known for its ability to support the lymphatic system, cleanse the blood, and promote hormonal balance. It is often used to support women's health, particularly during menopause, due to its mild estrogenic properties.

- Healing Properties: Supports the lymphatic system, cleanses the blood, promotes hormonal balance.
- How to Use: Red clover can be used in teas, tinctures, or added to salads for its nourishing and detoxifying benefits.

Guided Meditation:

- Sit comfortably and close your eyes. Visualize a field of red clover blooming under the sun, each flower radiating energy of gentle nourishment. As you inhale, feel this energy moving through your body, supporting your lymphatic system and cleansing your blood. With each exhale, release any toxins, allowing red clover to bring balance and vitality to your body.

Daily Ritual:

- Red Clover Tea for Lymphatic Support: Brew a cup of red clover tea to support your lymphatic system and promote gentle detoxification. As you drink, focus on how the herb helps your body cleanse and restore balance, particularly in your hormonal or lymphatic health.

Alternative Uses:

- Culinary Use: Add red clover blossoms to your salads for a mild, sweet taste that supports lymphatic health and hormonal balance.
- Tincture: Take red clover tincture daily to gently cleanse the blood and support the lymphatic system.
- Topical Use: Apply a red clover infusion as a wash for skin irritations or to promote skin healing.

XVI

Journaling Prompt:

What areas of your health feel stagnant or out of balance? How can you nourish your body to promote healing and vitality? Reflect on how red clover can help restore harmony in your physical and emotional body.

Day 16: Nettles (Urtica dioica)

Herb of the Day: Nettles

Nettles are a deeply nourishing and mineral-rich herb known for their ability to strengthen the body, support joint health, and reduce inflammation. Often called a "superfood" in the herbal world, nettles are an excellent herb for overall health and vitality.

- Healing Properties: Reduces inflammation, strengthens the body, supports joint health, and is rich in vitamins and minerals.
- How to Use: Nettles can be consumed as a tea, infusion, or used in cooking. They are also available in tincture form for convenient use.

Guided Meditation:

- Close your eyes and take a deep breath in. Visualize a strong, vibrant patch of nettles growing in rich soil. With each inhale, imagine the strength and vitality of the nettles filling your body, bringing nourishment to your muscles and bones. As you exhale, release any tension or inflammation, allowing the herb's energy to support your physical well-being.

Daily Ritual:

- Nettle Infusion for Vitality: Make a nettle infusion by steeping dried nettles in hot water for several hours. As you drink, focus on the rich, nourishing energy of the herb replenishing your body's minerals and supporting your overall health.

Alternative Uses:

- Culinary Use: Cook with fresh nettles by steaming or sautéing them to neutralize their sting, and add them to soups, stews, or stir-fries for a nutritious boost.
- Topical Use: Use nettle-infused oil or salve on sore joints or muscles to reduce inflammation and pain.
- Tincture: Take nettle tincture daily to support overall health, especially for joint health and reducing inflammation.

XVII

Journaling Prompt:

Where in your life do you need more strength or support? How can you nourish yourself to build that strength? Reflect on how nettles can help you restore vitality and fortify your body and mind.

Day 17: Elderflower (Sambucus nigra)

Herb of the Day: Elderflower

Elderflower is a gentle, soothing herb known for its ability to support respiratory health, reduce fever, and strengthen the immune system. Often used during colds and flu, elderflower is an excellent ally for seasonal changes and supporting overall wellness.

- Healing Properties: Supports respiratory health, reduces fever, strengthens the immune system.
- How to Use: Elderflower can be used in teas, tinctures, or as a syrup to support respiratory health and the immune system.

Guided Meditation:

- Close your eyes and take a deep breath, imagining the soft, fragrant elderflowers blooming in the early spring. With each inhale, feel the gentle, healing energy of elderflower entering your body, clearing your lungs and strengthening your immune system. As you exhale, let go of any tension or illness, allowing elderflower's energy to soothe and protect you.

Daily Ritual:

- Elderflower Tea for Respiratory Support: Brew a cup of elderflower tea to support your respiratory system and boost your immune health. As you sip, focus on how the gentle energy of the herb helps clear your lungs and protect your body from seasonal illnesses.

Alternative Uses:

- Syrup: Make elderflower syrup by simmering the flowers with honey, water, and lemon to create a delicious and immune-boosting syrup that can be taken daily.
- Tincture: Use elderflower tincture during cold and flu season to support respiratory health and reduce symptoms.
- Topical Use: Use elderflower as a wash for skin irritations or to reduce inflammation.

XVIII

Journaling Prompt:

How can you support your immune system and overall wellness? What areas of your health need extra attention during seasonal changes? Reflect on how elderflower's gentle, protective energy can help you stay healthy and resilient.

Day 18: Thyme (Thymus vulgaris)

Herb of the Day: Thyme

Thyme is a powerful antimicrobial herb known for its ability to support the respiratory system, fight infections, and boost the immune system. Its strong yet gentle energy makes it an excellent ally during cold and flu season, as well as for overall immune support.

- Healing Properties: Supports the respiratory system, fights infections, boosts the immune system, and is antimicrobial.
- How to Use: Thyme can be used in teas, tinctures, and as a culinary herb to support respiratory health and the immune system.

Guided Meditation:

- Close your eyes and take a deep breath in, imagining the sharp, fresh scent of thyme filling your lungs. With each inhale, feel the protective, cleansing energy of thyme supporting your respiratory system and boosting your immune defenses. As you exhale, let go of any lingering illness or tension, allowing thyme's energy to cleanse and fortify your body.

Daily Ritual:

- Thyme Steam for Respiratory Health: Boil water and add fresh or dried thyme to the pot. Place a towel over your head and lean over the pot, inhaling the thyme-infused steam to clear your lungs and sinuses. This ritual helps open airways and strengthen your respiratory system.

Alternative Uses:

- Culinary Use: Add fresh thyme to soups, stews, or roasted vegetables to enhance flavor while supporting your immune system.
- Tincture: Take a few drops of thyme tincture in water or tea when you feel a cold coming on or to support respiratory health during seasonal changes.
- Essential Oil: Dilute thyme essential oil in a carrier oil and massage into the chest or throat to relieve congestion and support respiratory function.

XIX

Journaling Prompt:

How can you strengthen your immune system and prepare for seasonal changes? Reflect on how you can protect your body from illness and boost your respiratory health, with thyme as a protective and cleansing ally.

Day 19: Skullcap (Scutellaria lateriflora)

erb of the Day: Skullcap

Skullcap is a gentle but powerful herb used to support the nervous system, relieve anxiety, and reduce muscle tension. It is an excellent herb for those looking to calm racing thoughts and bring a sense of peace to both body and mind.

- Healing Properties: Calms anxiety, relieves muscle tension, promotes restful sleep, supports the nervous system.
- How to Use: Skullcap can be consumed as a tea, tincture, or in capsule form for its calming effects on the mind and body.

Guided Meditation:

- Sit quietly and take a deep breath, feeling the soothing energy of skullcap entering your body. With each inhale, imagine the herb gently calming your nervous system and relaxing any areas of tension in your muscles. As you exhale, let go of stress, worry, or tightness, allowing skullcap to bring peace to your mind and body.

Daily Ritual:

- Skullcap Tea for Nervous System Support: Brew a cup of skullcap tea to calm your nerves and relieve muscle tension. As you drink, focus on how the herb soothes your body and mind, promoting relaxation and calm.

Alternative Uses:

- Tincture: Take skullcap tincture during moments of stress or anxiety to calm your mind and support your nervous system.
- Aromatherapy: Use skullcap-infused oil in a massage to relieve muscle tension and promote relaxation.
- Topical Use: Apply skullcap oil to tense muscles or areas of the body that feel tight or sore.

XX

Journaling Prompt:

Where do you hold tension in your body, and how can you release it? Reflect on how skullcap's calming energy can help you relax and let go of physical and mental tension.

Day 20: Valerian (Valeriana officinalis)

Herb of the Day: Valerian

Valerian is a powerful herb known for its sedative effects, making it a favorite for those struggling with insomnia, anxiety, or restlessness. While strong in its actions, valerian is gentle in its ability to calm the nervous system and promote deep, restful sleep.

- Healing Properties: Promotes restful sleep, calms anxiety, soothes restlessness.
- How to Use: Valerian is best used as a tea, tincture, or capsule to support sleep and reduce anxiety.

Guided Meditation:

- Close your eyes and take a deep breath in, focusing on the slow, calming energy of valerian. As you inhale, imagine valerian's sedative energy gently wrapping around you, easing any tension or restlessness in your body. With each exhale, release any lingering anxiety, allowing your body to fully relax and prepare for rest.

Daily Ritual:

- Valerian Tea for Sleep: Brew a cup of valerian tea before bed to support deep, restful sleep. As you drink, focus on how the herb calms your mind and prepares your body for a peaceful night of rest.

Alternative Uses:

- Tincture: Take valerian tincture in the evening to reduce anxiety and promote restful sleep.
- Aromatherapy: Use valerian essential oil in a diffuser to create a calming, sleep-inducing atmosphere in your bedroom.
- Topical Use: Dilute valerian essential oil in a carrier oil and massage into the back of your neck or temples to promote relaxation and relieve tension.

XXI

Journaling Prompt:

How can you create more restful moments in your life, both during the day and at night? Reflect on how valerian's calming energy can help you create space for rest and relaxation.

Day 21: Catnip (Nepeta cataria)

Herb of the Day: Catnip

While commonly known for its effect on cats, catnip is a wonderful herb for humans as well, particularly for calming the nerves and soothing the digestive system. It is gentle and safe, making it a great choice for both adults and children seeking relief from stress, anxiety, or digestive discomfort.

- Healing Properties: Calms the nerves, supports digestion, relieves stress and anxiety.
- How to Use: Catnip can be consumed as tea, tincture, or used topically to soothe anxiety and digestive issues.

Guided Meditation:

- Sit comfortably, close your eyes, and take a deep breath in. Imagine yourself in a peaceful garden surrounded by catnip plants. With each inhale, feel the calming, gentle energy of the herb entering your body, soothing any anxiety or stress. As you exhale, release any digestive discomfort or tension in your body, allowing catnip's calming influence to bring you peace.

Daily Ritual:

- Catnip Tea for Relaxation: Brew a cup of catnip tea when you're feeling anxious or stressed. As you sip, focus on how the herb calms your nerves and brings relaxation to both your mind and body.

Alternative Uses:

- Topical Use: Use catnip-infused oil to massage your abdomen and relieve digestive discomfort or cramps.
- Tincture: Take a few drops of catnip tincture to calm anxiety or nervous tension, especially during stressful moments.
- Aromatherapy: Diffuse catnip essential oil to create a calming environment that supports relaxation and stress relief.

XXII

Journaling Prompt:

What is currently causing you stress or anxiety, and how can you bring more calm into your life? Reflect on how catnip's soothing energy can help you reduce stress and bring more peace into your daily routine.

Day 22: Frankincense (Boswellia serrata)

erb of the Day: Frankincense

Frankincense is a resin known for its powerful anti-inflammatory and spiritual properties. It has been used for centuries in meditation and religious ceremonies to enhance spiritual connection and cleanse spaces. It also supports the immune system and reduces inflammation.

- Healing Properties: Reduces inflammation, supports the immune system, enhances spiritual connection.
- How to Use: Frankincense is commonly used in essential oils for aromatherapy or applied topically for inflammation relief.

Guided Meditation:

- Sit quietly and close your eyes. Imagine the calming, sacred scent of frankincense filling the air around you. With each inhale, feel the spiritual energy of the herb cleansing your mind and body. As you exhale, release any negative energy, allowing frankincense to bring a sense of peace and connection to your spiritual self.

Daily Ritual:

- Frankincense Aromatherapy for Spiritual Connection: Diffuse frankincense essential oil during meditation or quiet moments to enhance your spiritual awareness. Focus on how the scent calms your mind and deepens your connection to the present moment.

Alternative Uses:

- Topical Use: Dilute frankincense essential oil in a carrier oil and apply to areas of inflammation or joint pain to reduce swelling and promote healing.
- Incense: Burn frankincense resin as incense to cleanse your space and create a peaceful atmosphere.
- Aromatherapy: Inhale frankincense essential oil to support immune health and reduce inflammation.

XXIII

Journaling Prompt

How can you deepen your spiritual practice? Reflect on how frankincense's calming, sacred energy can help you connect with your higher self and promote peace in your life.

Day 23: Comfrey (Symphytum officinale)

H erb of the Day: Comfrey

Comfrey is a powerful herb used for healing bones, wounds, and skin issues. Known as "knitbone," comfrey promotes rapid cell regeneration, making it an excellent choice for healing injuries and promoting tissue repair.

- Healing Properties: Promotes bone and wound healing, supports skin regeneration, reduces inflammation.
- How to Use: Comfrey is best used topically in salves, poultices, or oils to promote wound healing and support tissue repair.

Guided Meditation:

- Close your eyes and take a deep breath in, imagining the healing energy of comfrey flowing through your body. With each inhale, visualize any areas of injury or tension in your body being soothed and regenerated. As you exhale, release any discomfort, allowing comfrey's healing properties to support your body's natural repair process.

Daily Ritual:

- Comfrey Salve for Healing: Apply comfrey salve to any cuts, scrapes, or sore muscles. As you massage it in, focus on how the herb promotes rapid healing and reduces inflammation in your body.

Alternative Uses:

- Poultice: Create a comfrey poultice by mashing fresh leaves and applying them to bruises, sprains, or sore muscles to promote healing.
- Infused Oil: Use comfrey-infused oil to massage into areas of injury, joint pain, or inflammation.
- Herbal Bath: Add comfrey leaves to a warm bath to soothe sore muscles and promote healing of the skin.

XXIV

Journaling Prompt:

*Where in your life or body do you need healing?
Reflect on how comfrey's ability to promote repair
and regeneration can support you in physical and
emotional healing.*

Day 24: Ashwagandha (Withania somnifera)

Herb of the Day: Ashwagandha

Ashwagandha is a powerful adaptogen known for its ability to reduce stress, support adrenal health, and increase energy levels. It is often used in Ayurvedic medicine to promote balance and vitality, particularly in times of physical or emotional stress.

- Healing Properties: Reduces stress, supports adrenal health, increases energy, promotes balance.
- How to Use: Ashwagandha can be consumed as a powder, in teas, or as a tincture to support overall vitality and stress management.

Guided Meditation:

- Sit quietly and close your eyes. Imagine the grounding energy of ashwagandha spreading through your body, bringing strength and resilience to every cell. With each inhale, feel yourself becoming more centered and balanced. As you exhale, release any stress or tension, allowing ashwagandha to bring peace and vitality to your body and mind.

Daily Ritual:

- Ashwagandha Tea for Stress Relief: Brew a cup of ashwagandha tea when you feel overwhelmed or fatigued. As you sip, focus on how the herb supports your body's ability to manage stress and increases your resilience.

Alternative Uses:

- Powder: Add ashwagandha powder to smoothies or warm milk to support adrenal health and reduce stress.
- Tincture: Take ashwagandha tincture daily to support overall vitality and reduce the effects of stress on your body.
- Capsules: Use ashwagandha capsules as a convenient way to incorporate the herb into your daily routine for stress management and energy support.

XXV

Journaling Prompt:

What areas of your life cause you the most stress, and how can you bring more balance into those spaces? Reflect on how ashwagandha's adaptogenic properties can help you manage stress and promote resilience.

Day 25: Black Cohosh (Actaea racemosa)

Herb of the Day: Black Cohosh

Black Cohosh is commonly used to support women's health, particularly for balancing hormones during menopause or menstrual cycles. It is known for its ability to relieve hot flashes, mood swings, and other symptoms related to hormonal imbalance.

- Healing Properties: Balances hormones, supports women's health, relieves menopausal and menstrual symptoms.
- How to Use: Black cohosh is typically consumed in tinctures, capsules, or teas to support hormonal balance and relieve menopausal symptoms.

Guided Meditation:

- Close your eyes and take a deep breath, focusing on the balancing energy of black cohosh. As you inhale, feel the herb's ability to bring harmony to your hormonal system. With each exhale, release any discomfort, mood swings, or tension related to your hormonal cycle.

Daily Ritual:

- Black Cohosh Tea for Hormonal Balance: Brew a cup of black cohosh tea to support hormonal balance, particularly during menopause or your menstrual cycle. As you sip, focus on how the herb helps to relieve symptoms and restore balance in your body.

Alternative Uses:

- Tincture: Take black cohosh tincture during menopause or your menstrual cycle to balance hormones and relieve symptoms such as hot flashes and mood swings.
- Capsules: Use black cohosh capsules daily to support women's health and maintain hormonal balance.
- Topical Use: Apply black cohosh-infused oil to areas of cramping or discomfort to promote relaxation and ease pain.

XXVI

Journaling Prompt:

How do your hormones affect your emotional and physical well-being? Reflect on how black cohosh's balancing properties can help you find harmony and ease during times of hormonal change.

Day 26: Garlic (Allium sativum)

Herb of the Day: Garlic

Garlic is a powerful antimicrobial and immune-boosting herb, used for centuries to fight infections and improve cardiovascular health. It is a staple in many natural remedies due to its ability to fight bacteria, fungi, and viruses.

- Healing Properties: Fights infections, boosts the immune system, improves cardiovascular health.
- How to Use: Garlic can be consumed raw, cooked, or in tinctures and capsules to support the immune system and fight infections.

Guided Meditation:

- Close your eyes and take a deep breath, imagining the strong, protective energy of garlic surrounding your body. With each inhale, feel garlic's immune-boosting properties strengthening your defenses. As you exhale, release any illness or weakness, allowing garlic's protective energy to fortify your health.

Daily Ritual:

- Garlic Tincture for Immune Support: Take garlic tincture when you feel a cold or infection coming on. As you take it, focus on how the herb fights off infections and strengthens your immune system.

Alternative Uses:

- Raw Garlic: Add raw garlic to your meals for its immune-boosting properties, or eat it directly for a more potent effect.
- Topical Use: Apply garlic-infused oil to areas of infection or fungal growth to fight bacteria and promote healing.
- Capsules: Use garlic capsules as a convenient way to boost your immune system daily.

XXVII

Journaling Prompt:

*How can you support your immune system and
protect your body from illness? Reflect on how garlic's
powerful energy can help you fortify your health and
fight off infections.*

Day 27: Hibiscus (Hibiscus sabdariffa)

Herb of the Day: Hibiscus

Hibiscus is a vibrant, cooling herb known for its ability to support heart health, reduce blood pressure, and provide antioxidant protection. Its tart, fruity flavor makes it a refreshing addition to teas, and it's often used to promote healthy circulation and cardiovascular health.

- Healing Properties: Supports heart health, lowers blood pressure, provides antioxidant protection.
- How to Use: Hibiscus can be enjoyed as a tea, tincture, or added to culinary dishes for its health benefits.

Guided Meditation:

- Close your eyes and take a deep breath in, imagining the vibrant red flowers of the hibiscus plant. With each inhale, feel the cooling, heart-strengthening energy of hibiscus entering your body. As you exhale, release any tension or stress, allowing the herb to bring peace and vitality to your heart.

Daily Ritual:

- Hibiscus Tea for Heart Health: Brew a cup of hibiscus tea, enjoying its tart, refreshing flavor. As you drink, focus on how the herb supports your heart and circulation, helping to lower blood pressure and promote overall cardiovascular health.

Alternative Uses:

- Culinary Use: Add dried hibiscus flowers to salads or desserts for a tart, fruity flavor that provides antioxidant protection.
- Tincture: Take hibiscus tincture daily to support heart health and lower blood pressure.
- Cold Infusion: Make a refreshing hibiscus cold infusion by steeping the flowers in cold water overnight, creating a hydrating, heart-healthy drink.

XXVIII

Journaling Prompt:

How can you better support your heart, both physically and emotionally? Reflect on how hibiscus can help you bring more care and vitality to your heart health.

Day 28: Rose Hips (Rosa canina)

Herb of the Day: Rose Hips

Rose hips, the fruit of the wild rose plant, are rich in vitamin C and antioxidants, making them excellent for boosting the immune system and supporting skin health. Their tart, citrusy flavor pairs well in teas and syrups, providing nourishment and protection for the body.

- Healing Properties: Boosts the immune system, supports skin health, provides antioxidants.
- How to Use: Rose hips can be consumed as a tea, syrup, or in tinctures for their immune-boosting and skin-supporting properties.

Guided Meditation:

- Sit comfortably and close your eyes, imagining a field of wild roses with vibrant red rose hips growing. As you inhale, feel the nourishing energy of rose hips filling your body with vitality and protection. With each exhale, release any illness or stress, allowing rose hips to strengthen and fortify your immune system.

Daily Ritual:

- Rose Hip Tea for Immunity: Brew a cup of rose hip tea, enjoying its tart, citrusy flavor. As you drink, focus on how the herb boosts your immune system and provides antioxidants to nourish and protect your body.

Alternative Uses:

- Syrup: Make a rose hip syrup to use as a topping for pancakes or mix with warm water for a vitamin C-rich tonic.
- Topical Use: Use rose hip-infused oil to promote skin health, especially for scars, wrinkles, or dry skin.
- Tincture: Take rose hip tincture daily to support immune function and overall vitality.

XXIX

Journaling Prompt:

How can you nourish and protect your body from illness and stress? Reflect on how rose hips can help you strengthen your immune system and support your overall well-being.

Day 29: Milk Thistle (Silybum marianum)

Herb of the Day: Milk Thistle

Milk Thistle is one of the most well-known herbs for liver support, helping to detoxify and protect the liver from toxins. It's a powerful herb used to promote overall detoxification, support liver function, and promote healthy skin.

- Healing Properties: Supports liver health, detoxifies the body, promotes skin health.
- How to Use: Milk thistle is commonly consumed as a tea, tincture, or capsule to support liver detoxification and overall health.

Guided Meditation:

- Close your eyes and imagine the protective energy of milk thistle wrapping around your liver, gently cleansing and detoxifying it. With each inhale, feel the herb supporting and strengthening your liver. As you exhale, release any toxins or stress, allowing milk thistle's protective energy to renew and restore your body.

Daily Ritual:

- Milk Thistle Tea for Detoxification: Brew a cup of milk thistle tea to support liver health and detoxification. As you drink, focus on how the herb cleanses your liver and promotes overall health and vitality.

Alternative Uses:

- Capsules: Take milk thistle capsules daily to support liver detoxification and protect the liver from toxins.
- Tincture: Use milk thistle tincture to promote liver health and overall detoxification.
- Topical Use: Use milk thistle-infused oil on the skin to promote healing and detoxification, particularly for acne or skin irritation.

XXX

Journaling Prompt:

What areas of your life or body need detoxification or cleansing? Reflect on how milk thistle's detoxifying properties can help you release toxins and restore balance in your life.

Day 30: Slippery Elm (Ulmus rubra)

Herb of the Day: Slippery Elm

Slippery Elm is a soothing and mucilaginous herb known for its ability to support digestive health, soothe inflammation, and ease sore throats. It forms a protective coating on mucous membranes, making it especially beneficial for those with gastrointestinal or respiratory issues.

- Healing Properties: Soothes the digestive tract, reduces inflammation, supports respiratory health.
- How to Use: Slippery Elm is most often consumed as a powder mixed with water to create a mucilaginous drink, or used in lozenges for throat relief.

Guided Meditation:

- Close your eyes and imagine a soft, protective layer enveloping your throat and stomach, easing any discomfort. As you inhale, feel the soothing energy of slippery elm calming any inflammation or irritation in your body. As you exhale, let go of any physical or emotional discomfort, allowing the herb to bring you peace and ease.

Daily Ritual:

- Slippery Elm Tea for Digestive Health: Mix slippery elm powder with warm water to create a soothing tea. As you sip, focus on how the herb coats and protects your digestive system, easing any inflammation or irritation.

Alternative Uses:

- Lozenges: Use slippery elm lozenges to soothe sore throats and support respiratory health.
- Topical Use: Make a slippery elm poultice by mixing the powder with water and applying it to irritated skin or wounds to promote healing.
- Tincture: Use slippery elm tincture to soothe digestive discomfort and support gut health.

XXXI

Journaling Prompt:

Where in your life or body do you feel irritation or discomfort? How can you bring more ease and protection to those areas? Reflect on how slippery elm's soothing energy can support your well-being.

Bonus Day 31: English Ivy (Hedera helix)

Herb of the Day: English Ivy

English Ivy is known for its respiratory support, particularly for clearing congestion and easing coughs. It has been used for centuries to treat bronchial conditions, and its ability to soothe the respiratory system makes it a valuable herb for lung health and overall respiratory well-being.

- Healing Properties: Supports respiratory health, reduces congestion, soothes coughs.
- How to Use: English ivy is commonly used as a tea, tincture, or in syrups for respiratory support.

Guided Meditation:

- Close your eyes and take a deep breath in, imagining the protective vines of English ivy wrapping gently around your lungs. As you inhale, feel the herb clearing your airways and easing any tension in your chest. With each exhale, release any congestion or discomfort, allowing English ivy's energy to bring ease to your breathing.

Daily Ritual:

• English Ivy Tea for Respiratory Health: Brew a cup of English ivy tea to support your lungs and ease any coughs or congestion. As you drink, focus on how the herb opens your airways and clears away blockages, bringing fresh energy to your respiratory system.

Alternative Uses:

• Syrup: Make an English ivy syrup to use as a natural remedy for coughs and respiratory irritation.
• Tincture: Take English ivy tincture to soothe the lungs and support respiratory health, especially during colds or flu.
• Topical Use: Use an ivy-infused salve or ointment to soothe irritated skin or insect bites.

XXXII

Journaling Prompt:

How can you support your respiratory health and bring more breath into your life? Reflect on how English ivy's ability to clear congestion and soothe the lungs can help you breathe easier, both physically and emotionally.

Conclusion

Reflecting on Your Journey

As you reach the end of The Modern Herbalist's Guide: 30 Days to Healing and Harmony, take a moment to reflect on the journey you've completed. Over the last month, you've connected with powerful herbs, established mindful rituals, and embraced the healing energy of nature. Each herb has supported you in a different way—whether by easing stress, boosting your immune system, or promoting emotional balance.

Remember that healing is an ongoing process, and these herbs and practices are here to support you whenever you need them. Continue to integrate the rituals you've learned into your daily life, and know that nature's wisdom is always available to you.

Take a deep breath and feel gratitude for this journey of self-care and healing. You've taken important steps toward nurturing your body, mind, and spirit, and this is just the beginning.

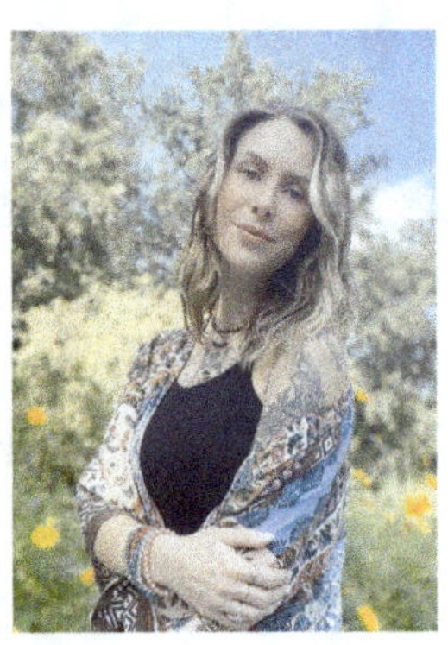

About the Author

Samantha Peterein is the founder of Luna & Daisy Herbal Co. LLC, a woman-owned small business located in rural Missouri. As a passionate herbalist and healer, Samantha is devoted to understanding the profound connection between nature and wellness. She has completed studies in herbalism, natural and herbal medicine, naturopathy, and Ayurvedic herbal medicine, bringing both depth and breadth to her practice.

With a deep calling to nurture and heal, Samantha shares her gifts with the world through her small business and her writings. As a wife and mother, she knows firsthand the importance of balance, self-care, and supporting the well-being of those we love. Her mission is to empower others to embrace natural remedies and rituals, making holistic healing accessible and approachable for everyone.

Through Luna & Daisy Herbal Co., Samantha brings her personal journey of healing and her knowledge of herbs to her community and beyond. Her work is grounded in compassion, intuition, and a desire to help others rediscover the healing power of nature. Samantha continues to share her wisdom, offering tools and guidance for those seeking to restore harmony in their body, mind, and spirit.

You can connect with me on:

🌐 https://www.lunaanddaisyherbalcollc.com